Conquering Thyroid Cancer

An Ultimate Guide to Treatment, Recovery, and Thriving After Diagnosis

Isabella White

Copyright © 2023 by Isabella White.

Disclaimer: The information contained in this book is based on the research, opinions, and experiences of the author. It is not intended to replace professional medical advice or treatment. The reader should regularly consult a physician for any health issues and always seek the advice of a physician before modifying diet, supplement, or exercise regimens.

The author and publisher shall have neither liability nor responsibility to any person or entity concerning any loss or damage related to the information contained in this book. The information provided is general in nature and may not apply to every individual. Any reliance on the information contained herein is solely at the reader's own risk.

Contents

Introduction

Thyroid cancer is a type of cancer that affects the thyroid gland, which is a little butterfly-shaped gland in the front of the neck. The thyroid gland serves a crucial role in controlling the metabolism of the body and releasing hormones that affect various biological functions.

Thyroid cancer develops when abnormal cells in the thyroid gland begin to grow and divide uncontrollably, resulting in the formation of a tumor. While the actual origin of thyroid cancer is unknown, various risk factors, such as radiation exposure, a family history of thyroid cancer, and certain genetic abnormalities, have been found.

Thyroid cancer is uncommon in comparison to other types of cancer, but its prevalence has been progressively rising over the last few decades. It affects people between the ages of 30 and 60, and it is more common in women than in men.

Thyroid cancer is classified into various types, each with its own set of characteristics and treatment options. The most common types are as follows:

Papillary thyroid cancer: This is the most common type of thyroid cancer, accounting for about 80% of cases. It develops slowly and has a high cure rate.

Follicular thyroid cancer: This type accounts for approximately 10–15% of cases and spreads to other parts of the body more frequently than papillary thyroid cancer.

Medullary thyroid cancer: This type accounts for roughly 4% of cases and arises from the thyroid gland's C cells. It might be inherited or sporadic.

Anaplastic thyroid cancer: This is the rarest and most aggressive type of thyroid cancer, accounting for less than 2% of cases. It grows and spreads quickly, making treatment more challenging.

Thyroid cancer is often categorized into stages based on tumor size, whether it has spread to nearby lymph nodes, and whether it has metastasized to other parts of the body. The staging method helps assess each individual's most effective therapy approach and prognosis.

Early-stage thyroid cancer is frequently asymptomatic, which means there are no visible signs or symptoms. A lump or enlargement in the neck, trouble swallowing or breathing, hoarseness, a persistent cough, and unexplained weight loss are all common symptoms of cancer as it develops.

Thyroid cancer is typically diagnosed using a combination of physical examination, imaging tests (such as ultrasound, CT scan, or MRI), blood tests, and a biopsy. The most conclusive method of confirming the existence of cancer cells in the thyroid gland is a biopsy.

Once a thyroid cancer diagnosis has been made, a multidisciplinary team of healthcare specialists, including endocrinologists, surgeons, radiation oncologists, and medical oncologists, will collaborate to design a personalized treatment plan.

Thyroid cancer treatment options include surgery, radioactive iodine therapy, external beam radiation therapy, chemotherapy, and targeted therapy. The type and stage of the cancer, as well as the patient's overall health and preferences, will determine the precise treatment options.

Significant advances in thyroid cancer treatment have been made in recent years, resulting in improved patient outcomes and quality of life. The prognosis for thyroid cancer is generally favorable, with a high survival rate, given early discovery and effective treatment.

We will delve deeper into the various aspects of thyroid cancer in the following sections of this book, including its causes and risk factors, diagnosis and screening methods, treatment options, recovery and rehabilitation strategies, long-term follow-up and monitoring, and tips for thriving after thyroid cancer.

We will also share the inspirational experiences of thyroid cancer survivors who have successfully navigated their journey, as well as practical tips on how to develop a support network and manage the emotional and psychological aspects of living with thyroid cancer.

Chapter 1

Understanding Thyroid Cancer

Types and Stages of Thyroid Cancer

Thyroid cancer is an uncommon type of cancer that affects the thyroid gland, which is a little butterfly-shaped gland in the front of the neck. This gland plays a crucial role in regulating the metabolism of the body and releasing hormones that are essential for various biological activities. Understanding the various types and stages of thyroid cancer is important for both patients and healthcare providers to determine the best treatment plan and prognosis.

Types of Thyroid Cancer

There are various types of thyroid cancer, each with unique characteristics and treatment approaches. The most common types are as follows:

Papillary Thyroid Cancer (PTC): PTC is the most common type of thyroid cancer, accounting for approximately 80% of all cases. PTC grows slowly and is frequently seen in one lobe of the thyroid gland. It has a high cure rate and primarily affects younger people, particularly women.

Follicular Thyroid Cancer (FTC): FTC accounts for around 10-15% of thyroid cancer cases. It typically affects people over the age of 40 and is more common in locations where iodine levels are low. When compared to PTC, FTC has a higher chance of spreading to distant organs.

Medullary Thyroid Cancer (MTC): MTC develops from the thyroid gland's C cells, which produce the hormone calcitonin. It accounts for around 4% of all thyroid cancer cases. MTC can be hereditary or sporadic, with the hereditary variety frequently accompanied by other endocrine challenges. Individuals with MTC should undergo genetic testing to determine if the condition is hereditary.

Anaplastic Thyroid Cancer (ATC): ATC is a rare and severe kind of thyroid cancer, accounting for fewer than 2% of cases. It is more common in older people and has a dismal prognosis. ATC develops quickly and can infiltrate nearby structures, making treatment difficult.

Thyroid Lymphoma: Thyroid lymphoma is a rare type of thyroid cancer that develops from lymphocytes, a type of white blood cell. It accounts for less than 2% of cases of thyroid cancer. Thyroid lymphoma is more common in older people and could appear as a quickly developing lump in the neck.

Stages of Thyroid Cancer

Thyroid cancer is staged based on tumor size, the extent of spread to nearby lymph nodes or other organs, and if it has metastasized (spread) to distant sites in the body. The American Joint Committee on Cancer (AJCC) TNM classification is the most generally used staging method for thyroid cancer. The stages are numbered I through IV, with subcategories within each.

- **Stage I:** The tumor is restricted to the thyroid gland and is less than 2 centimeters (cm) in size. It has not spread to the lymph nodes or other distant sites.
- **Stage II:** The tumor has grown to be more than 2 centimeters (cm) in size but is still confined to the thyroid gland. It has not spread to the lymph nodes or other distant sites.
- **Stage III:** The tumor has spread to surrounding lymph nodes or structures such as the trachea, esophagus, or larynx. It may or may not have spread to distant sites.
- **Stage IV:** This stage is divided into two subcategories:

  a. Stage IVA: The tumor has spread beyond the thyroid gland and has infiltrated surrounding structures, including the trachea, esophagus, or blood vessels. It could have spread to lymph nodes or not.

b. Stage IVB: The tumor has spread to the lymph nodes in the neck or to distant sites in the body, such as the lungs or bones.

c. Stage IVC: The tumor has spread to distant sites within the body, such as the lungs, liver, or bones.

It is important to highlight that the thyroid cancer stage is only one element in deciding prognosis and treatment options. Other criteria, such as the type of thyroid cancer, the patient's age and overall health, and the existence of genetic alterations, also play a role in treatment decisions.

In a nutshell, both patients and healthcare providers must understand the various kinds and stages of thyroid cancer. Each type of thyroid cancer has unique characteristics and treatment approaches, and the cancer's stage helps determine the extent of its spread and directs treatment decisions. Patients can actively engage in their treatment and make informed decisions about their care if they have a full understanding of the disease.

Causes and Risk Factors of Thyroid Cancer

Thyroid cancer is a type of cancer that affects the thyroid gland, a small butterfly-shaped gland at the base of the neck. The thyroid gland serves a crucial role in controlling the metabolism of the body and releasing hormones that affect various body functions. When cells in the thyroid gland begin to grow and divide uncontrolled, it can lead to the development of thyroid cancer.

While the precise etiology of thyroid cancer is unknown, experts have identified several risk factors that may increase a person's chances of developing the disease. It's important to note that having one or more risk factors does not guarantee that you'll get thyroid cancer.

Some people with thyroid cancer, on the other hand, may have no identified risk factors. However, understanding these health risk factors can help individuals make informed health decisions and take necessary measures for early detection and prevention.

Gender: Thyroid cancer is more common in women than in men. Women are three times more likely than men to have thyroid cancer. The cause of this gender disparity is unknown, but it may be related to hormonal factors.

Age: Thyroid cancer can develop at any age, but it is most typically detected in people aged 30 to 60. The risk of developing thyroid cancer increases with age, with individuals over the age of 60 having the greatest incidence rates.

Family History: Having a close family member with thyroid cancer, such as a parent or sibling, increases the risk of developing the condition. Individuals are additionally predisposed to thyroid cancer by certain hereditary genetic diseases, such as familial medullary thyroid cancer and multiple endocrine neoplasia type 2.

Radiation Exposure: Exposure to high levels of radiation, particularly during youth, is a well-known risk factor for thyroid cancer. This includes exposure through medical treatments such as head and neck radiation therapy as well as exposure from environmental sources such as nuclear accidents or radiation fallout.

Previous Thyroid Conditions: Individuals with a history of thyroid disorders such as goiter (enlarged thyroid gland), thyroid nodules, or thyroiditis (inflammation of the thyroid gland) have an increased risk of developing thyroid cancer. It is important to note that the majority of thyroid nodules and goiters are not malignant.

Iodine Deficiency or Excess: Iodine is an essential nutrient that is necessary for the formation of thyroid hormones. The risk of developing thyroid cancer can be increased by iodine deficiency as well as excess. This risk factor is less significant in countries where iodine shortages are uncommon due to iodized salt or other iodine sources.

Obesity: Some research has linked obesity to an increased risk of thyroid cancer, particularly in women. The precise mechanism underlying this relationship is unknown, but it could be related to hormonal changes and inflammation associated with obesity.

Certain Genetic Mutations: Certain genetic mutations, such as mutations in the BRAF or RET genes, have been linked to an increased risk of developing thyroid cancer. These mutations can be passed down through families or acquired during a person's lifetime.

It is important to remember that possessing one or more of these risk factors does not ensure the development of thyroid cancer. Individuals without known risk factors, on the other hand, can nonetheless get the disease.

Individuals should be cautious about their health, undertake frequent tests, and consult with healthcare specialists for proper evaluation and management if risk factors are present. The prognosis and results for individuals diagnosed with thyroid cancer can be greatly improved by early detection and treatment.

Diagnosis and Screening of Thyroid Cancer

Thyroid cancer is usually diagnosed using a combination of medical history, physical examination, and various diagnostic tests. In this section, we will look at several methods for diagnosing and screening thyroid cancer.

Physical Examination and Medical History

A comprehensive medical history and physical examination are the first steps in the diagnostic process when a patient appears with symptoms that may be indicative of thyroid cancer. The healthcare professional will inquire about the patient's symptoms, cancer family history, and any risk factors that may increase the possibility of thyroid cancer.

The healthcare professional will carefully inspect the neck area during the physical examination, feeling for any lumps or abnormalities in the thyroid gland. They may also look for swollen lymph nodes in the neck, which might be a sign that the cancer has spread.

Thyroid Function Tests

Thyroid function tests are blood tests used to measure the levels of thyroid hormones in the body. These tests are important in the diagnosis of thyroid cancer because certain types of thyroid cancer can interfere with the production of thyroid hormones.

The thyroid-stimulating hormone (TSH) test is the most often used thyroid function test. TSH levels that are elevated may indicate an underactive thyroid (hypothyroidism), which is an indication of thyroid cancer. Additionally, the thyroid gland may measure thyroglobulin levels. Elevated thyroglobulin levels might also be a sign of thyroid cancer.

Imaging Tests

Imaging tests are frequently performed to visualize the thyroid gland and surrounding structures, which help identify any abnormalities or tumors. The following are the most commonly utilized imaging tests for identifying thyroid cancer:

- **Ultrasound:** This non-invasive test creates images of the thyroid gland using sound waves. It can help determine the size, shape, and composition of any nodules or tumors that may be present.
- **Computed Tomography (CT) Scan:** A CT scan creates detailed cross-sectional images of the body using X-rays and computer technologies. It can provide information on the size and location of tumors, as well as if the cancer has spread to nearby lymph nodes or other organs.
- **Magnetic Resonance Imaging (MRI):** MRI creates detailed images of the body by using powerful magnets and radio waves. It is particularly helpful in determining the extent of tumor involvement and detecting any spread to surrounding structures.
- **Positron Emission Tomography (PET) Scan:** A PET scan involves the injection of a small amount of radioactive material into the body. Cancer cells absorb this substance, allowing a specific camera to spot them. PET scans are frequently used to determine

whether or not the cancer has spread to other parts of the body.

Fine Needle Aspiration (FNA) Biopsy

A tiny needle aspiration biopsy is a process in which cells are extracted from a suspected nodule or tumor in the thyroid gland using a thin needle. The cells are then analyzed under a microscope to determine their malignant status.

The FNA biopsy is the gold standard for diagnosing thyroid cancer. It is a reasonably straightforward and safe procedure that can be performed in the office of a healthcare provider. The biopsy results can help determine the type of thyroid cancer present and guide subsequent treatment decisions.

Other Diagnostic Tests

Additional diagnostic tests may be required in some cases to confirm a diagnosis or provide more information about the cancer. These tests may involve the following:

- **Thyroid scan:** This test involves the injection of a small amount of radioactive material into the body, which is then absorbed by the thyroid gland. A unique camera is then used to capture images of the thyroid, helping to identify any areas of aberrant activity.
- **Genetic testing:** For certain types of thyroid cancer, particularly if there is a family history of the disease, genetic testing may be recommended. These tests can

help identify specific gene mutations that may increase the risk of developing thyroid cancer.

- **Blood tests:** Other blood tests, in addition to thyroid function tests, may be performed to examine overall health and detect any abnormalities that may be related to thyroid cancer.

Screening for Thyroid Cancer

In contrast to several other types of cancer, there is currently no generally recommended screening test for thyroid cancer in individuals who do not have symptoms or risk factors. Thyroid cancer screening is not recommended for the general population.

Individuals with a family history of thyroid cancer or certain genetic abnormalities that increase the risk of developing the disease, on the other hand, may be advised to undergo regular screening. To monitor for any changes or abnormalities, this may entail periodic ultrasound examinations of the thyroid gland.

It is important to note that the benefits and limitations of thyroid cancer screening should be reviewed with a healthcare provider, taking individual risk factors and preferences into account.

In essence, thyroid cancer diagnosis entails a combination of medical history, physical examination, and various diagnostic tests. Thyroid function tests, imaging tests, a fine needle aspiration biopsy, and other diagnostic procedures are used to confirm the diagnosis of thyroid cancer and provide important information for treatment planning. While routine thyroid cancer screening is not recommended for the general population, individuals with a family history or particular risk factors may be advised to do so.

Chapter 2

Treatment Options for Thyroid Cancer

Surgery

One of the primary treatment options for thyroid cancer is surgery. Various surgical procedures involve the removal of cancerous thyroid tissue. The specific type of surgery recommended is determined by the size, location, and stage of the cancer, as well as the individual's overall health.

Types of Thyroid Surgery

Various types of thyroid surgery may be performed, including:

- **Total Thyroidectomy:** This procedure involves the removal of the entire thyroid gland. It is the most commonly used surgical approach in the treatment of thyroid cancer. Total thyroidectomy is frequently recommended for bigger tumors, aggressive forms of thyroid cancer, or when the risk of cancer recurrence is high.

- **Partial Thyroidectomy:** This surgery, also known as a lobectomy, involves the removal of only one lobe of the thyroid gland. It is usually performed when the cancer is confined to one side of the thyroid or when the tumor is tiny in size. Following a partial thyroidectomy, radioactive iodine therapy may be used to kill any remaining cancer cells.

- **Thyroidectomy (Near-Total):** This procedure involves the removal of practically the whole thyroid gland, leaving only a small quantity of thyroid tissue behind. When there is a concern about maintaining the parathyroid glands or the recurrent laryngeal nerves, which are important for regulating calcium levels and voice function, a near-total thyroidectomy may be recommended.

- **Subtotal Thyroidectomy:** A considerable amount of the thyroid gland is removed in this surgery, leaving only a small residual. Subtotal thyroidectomy is rarely performed nowadays, as total or near-total thyroidectomy has essentially replaced it.

Getting Prepared for Surgery

It's important to have a full talk with your healthcare team before undergoing thyroid surgery. They will explain the procedure, go over the risks and advantages, and address any concerns or questions you may have. Preoperative tests, such as blood tests, imaging scans, and a fine-needle aspiration biopsy, may also be performed to determine the extent and kind of the cancer.

Before surgery, your doctor may recommend thyroid hormone replacement treatment in some cases. This involves using synthetic thyroid hormone medication to decrease the synthesis of thyroid-stimulating hormone (TSH), which can accelerate the growth of thyroid cancer cells. By reducing TSH levels, surgery may be safer and more effective by slowing the growth of cancer.

The Surgical Procedure

Thyroid surgery is usually performed under general anesthesia, which means you will be sleeping throughout the procedure. To access the thyroid gland, the surgeon will make an incision in the front of your neck, usually along a natural skin crease. The size and location of the incision may vary according to the extent of the surgery and the surgeon's preference.

The surgeon will carefully remove the cancerous thyroid tissue, as well as any nearby lymph nodes that may be affected, during the surgery. The removed tissue will be sent to a pathology laboratory for further evaluation to determine the cancer's stage and characteristics.

In some cases, the surgeon may use intraoperative nerve monitoring to identify and protect the recurrent laryngeal nerves, which regulate vocal cord movement. This helps to reduce the risk of nerve damage and possibly voice alterations following surgery.

Potential Complications and Recovery

You will be closely watched in the recovery room following thyroid surgery before being transported to a hospital room or discharged home. The length of stay in the hospital may vary based on the extent of the surgery and individual factors.

Postoperative treatment commonly includes pain management, vital sign monitoring, and wound care. You may suffer some soreness, swelling, and bruising around the incision site, which can be managed with pain relievers and cold compresses.

Thyroid surgery complications are uncommon; however, they can include bleeding, infection, damage to the parathyroid glands or recurrent laryngeal nerves, and hypothyroidism. Hypothyroidism occurs when the thyroid gland fails to generate enough thyroid hormone, and it can be managed with lifelong thyroid hormone replacement treatment.

Follow-Up Care

Following surgery, you will have regular follow-up consultations with your healthcare team to monitor your recovery and evaluate the treatment's effectiveness. Physical examinations, blood tests to assess thyroid hormone levels, and imaging scans to detect any symptoms of recurrence or metastasis may be part of these consultations.

Based on the characteristics of the cancer and the necessity for additional treatment, your doctor may additionally propose radioactive iodine therapy or other adjuvant treatments.

Surgery plays a crucial role in the treatment of thyroid cancer, in conclusion. Depending on the extent and stage of the cancer, it involves the removal of malignant thyroid tissue and may be performed in various ways. While recovery from surgery may take some time, many individuals with thyroid cancer can lead healthy and productive lives with the right care and follow-up.

Radioactive Iodine Therapy

Radioactive iodine therapy, often known as RAI or radioactive iodine ablation, is a common treatment option for thyroid cancer. It involves the use of a radioactive type of iodine following surgery to eliminate any remaining thyroid tissue or cancer cells. This therapy is particularly effective at locating and eliminating cancer cells that may have spread outside of the thyroid gland.

What Is the Process of Radioactive Iodine Therapy?

Thyroid cells are the only cells in the body that can absorb and concentrate iodine; therefore, radioactive iodine therapy makes use of this feature. Thyroid hormones, which control various biological functions, are produced by the thyroid gland using iodine. The radiation is selectively picked up by any surviving thyroid tissue or cancer cells after injecting a radioactive type of iodine.

Once inside the thyroid cells, the radioactive iodine generates radiation that destroys the cells' DNA, ultimately leading to their destruction. The radiation also damages cancer cells nearby, which may have spread to lymph nodes or other parts of the body. The goal of radioactive iodine therapy is to eliminate any remaining cancer cells and reduce the risk of recurrence.

Who is a Candidate for Radioactive Iodine Therapy?

Thyroid cancer patients do not always require radioactive iodine therapy. The decision to proceed with this treatment is influenced by several factors, including the type and stage of the cancer, the presence of leftover thyroid tissue or cancer cells, and the risk of recurrence. Your healthcare team will assess your unique situation to determine if radioactive iodine therapy is right for you.

The following conditions are typically recommended for radioactive iodine therapy:

- **Patients with differentiated thyroid cancer:** Patients with papillary or follicular thyroid cancer, the two main types of differentiated thyroid cancer, are the most common candidates for radioactive iodine therapy. These cancers absorb iodine effectively and respond well to treatment.

- **Patients with high-risk features:** If your cancer has specific high-risk characteristics, such as large tumor size, lymph node spread, or invasion of blood vessels or surrounding tissues, your healthcare team may consider radioactive iodine therapy to reduce the risk of recurrence.

- **Patients with remaining thyroid tissue or cancer cells:** Small amounts of thyroid tissue or cancer cells may remain in the body after surgery to remove the thyroid gland (total thyroidectomy). Radioactive iodine therapy can help eliminate any residual cells.

What Can You Expect From Radioactive Iodine Therapy?
You must prepare for radioactive iodine therapy by following the instructions provided by your healthcare team. These guidelines may include the following:

- **Discontinuing certain medications:** Certain medications, such as thyroid hormone replacement therapy, may reduce the effectiveness of radioactive iodine therapy. When to discontinue taking these drugs will be determined by your healthcare team.

- **Following a low-iodine diet:** A low-iodine diet helps to deplete the body's iodine stores, making the thyroid cells more receptive to radioactive iodine. This diet often involves avoiding foods high in iodine, such as seafood, dairy products, and iodized salt.

- **Temporary isolation:** Due to the radioactivity of the treatment, you may need to stay in isolation for a short period. This is to protect people from unnecessary radiation exposure. Your healthcare team will provide specific advice on how long you should isolate yourself.

You will be given a pill or liquid containing radioactive iodine to swallow during the treatment. The radiation is subsequently taken up by thyroid and cancer cells. The amount of radiation you receive will be determined by your specific instance and the treatment's goal.

You may notice certain side effects after the treatment, such as dry mouth, changes in taste, or brief neck pain. These adverse effects are usually mild and will go away on their own. Your healthcare team will provide you with instructions on how to manage any discomfort or adverse effects.

Follow-Up and Monitoring After Radioactive Iodine Therapy

Following radioactive iodine therapy, you will need to meet with your healthcare team frequently to monitor your progress and assess the effectiveness of the treatment. Blood tests to measure thyroid hormone levels, imaging scans to assess treatment response, and physical examinations may be part of these consultations.

Additional doses of radioactive iodine therapy may be required in some cases if there is evidence of persistent or recurring disease. Based on your specific case, your healthcare team will determine the most effective course of action.

It is important to note that you may need to take thyroid hormone replacement medication for the rest of your life if you receive radioactive iodine therapy. This is because the hormones frequently lead to hypothyroidism (treatment), and the medication helps to replace the missing hormones.

Radioactive iodine therapy is a promising treatment option for patients with thyroid cancer, particularly those with differentiated thyroid cancer and high-risk characteristics. It successfully targets and eliminates residual thyroid tissue or cancer cells, lowering the risk of recurrence. You can achieve the best possible outcome from radioactive iodine therapy by following the directions provided by your healthcare team and attending regular follow-up sessions.

External Beam Radiation Therapy

External beam radiation therapy (EBRT) targets and destroys thyroid cancer cells using high-energy X-rays or protons. This type of radiation therapy is delivered from outside the body by a machine and is precisely aimed at the tumor spot. To effectively treat thyroid cancer, EBRT is frequently used in combination with other treatments such as surgery or radioactive iodine therapy.

How Does External Beam Radiation Therapy Work?

A radiation oncologist will carefully design and administer the treatment during external beam radiation therapy. Usually, the process involves the following steps:

- **Simulation:** Before starting the actual treatment, a simulation session is conducted to determine the precise area that needs to be treated. This involves using imaging tests such as CT scans or MRIs to build a thorough map of the tumor and surrounding structures. To ensure precision, the patient will be positioned exactly as they will be throughout treatment.

- **Treatment Planning:** The radiation oncologist will develop a treatment plan based on the information acquired during the simulation. The dosage, number of treatments, and angles at which the radiation beams will be delivered are all outlined in this plan. The goal is to increase the radiation dose to the tumor while limiting radiation exposure to healthy tissues.

- **Treatment Sessions:** For several weeks, treatment sessions are often planned every day, Monday through

Friday. Each session is brief, lasting only a few minutes. The radiation therapist will position the patient on a treatment table based on the marks made during the simulation. The radiation equipment will then administer radiation beams to the specified area.

- **Monitoring and follow-up:** The radiation oncology team will regularly monitor the patient's progress during treatment. To assess the tumor's response to radiation therapy, regular check-ups, and imaging scans may be conducted. Following completion of the treatment, the patient will be scheduled for follow-up consultations to monitor long-term recovery and manage any potential side effects.

Effectiveness of External Beam Radiation Therapy for Thyroid Cancer

For certain types and stages of thyroid cancer, external beam radiation therapy can be an effective treatment option. It is most commonly used in the following situations:

- **Adjuvant Therapy:** Following thyroid gland removal surgery (total thyroidectomy), EBRT may be recommended to destroy any leftover cancer cells in the neck area. This helps reduce recurrence risk.

- **Locally Advanced or Recurrent Cancer:** EBRT can be used to target and destroy cancer cells in cases where the cancer has spread to nearby tissues or has returned after initial treatment.

- **Palliative Care:** EBRT can be used to relieve symptoms and enhance the patient's quality of life in advanced cases of thyroid cancer where a cure is not achievable. It can help reduce tumors that are causing pain or other problems.

External Beam Radiation Therapy's Potential Side Effects

External beam radiation therapy might have side effects, just like any other medical treatment. The specific side effects felt may differ depending on the individual and the dosage of radiation administered. The following are common side effects of EBRT for thyroid cancer:

- **Skin Changes:** The treated area's skin may become red, dry, or irritated. It may grow more sensitive to sunlight in some cases. During and after treatment, it's important to take care of your skin and protect yourself from the sun.

- **Fatigue:** Many patients experience fatigue during radiation therapy. This can range from mild to severe, and it may persist for several weeks after treatment is complete. Resting, maintaining a healthy diet, and staying hydrated can all help manage fatigue.

- **Swallowing Difficulties:** Radiation therapy to the neck area can create temporary swallowing difficulties. This normally improves following treatment, but it may persist in certain cases. Working with a speech therapist or a dietician can help you manage swallowing problems.

- **Nausea and Vomiting:** Although rare, some patients may experience nausea and vomiting as a result of radiation therapy. To help manage these symptoms, medications can be provided.

- **Hair Loss:** Hair loss is not a common side effect of thyroid cancer treatment with EBRT. However, temporary hair loss may occur if the treatment area involves the scalp. Hair usually regrows within a few months of treatment.

It is important to note that not all patients will have these side effects, and the severity of these effects can vary. The radiation oncology team will continuously monitor the patient's progress and will provide supportive care to help manage any side effects that may occur.

External beam radiation therapy is an effective treatment for thyroid cancer. It can be used after surgery as an adjuvant therapy, to treat locally advanced or recurring cancer, or to provide palliative care. While there may be some side effects, they are generally controllable and transitory. The radiation oncology team will work closely with the patient to develop a specific treatment plan and will provide ongoing support throughout the process.

Chemotherapy and Targeted Therapy

Chemotherapy and targeted therapy are two additional thyroid cancer treatment options. While surgery, radioactive iodine therapy, and external beam radiation therapy are the most common treatment options, chemotherapy and targeted therapy may be recommended in some cases. In this section, we will look in depth at different treatment alternatives, including how they function, when they are used, and what potential side effects they may have.

Chemotherapy

Chemotherapy is a systemic treatment that uses drugs to either kill or restrict the growth of cancer cells. Chemotherapy spreads throughout the body, targeting cancer cells that may have spread beyond the thyroid gland, unlike surgery or radiation therapy, which targets specific places. It is usually given as an intravenous (IV) infusion or in the form of oral medicines.

Chemotherapy is not a common first-line treatment for thyroid cancer. It is often reserved for advanced or metastatic cases of cancer that have spread to other parts of the body. Chemotherapy may also be utilized in cases where other treatments have failed or if the cancer is not responsive to radioactive iodine therapy.

The specific chemotherapy drugs used to treat thyroid cancer can differ based on the type and stage of the cancer. Doxorubicin, cisplatin, and paclitaxel are among the most commonly utilized drugs. These drugs function by interfering with the ability of cancer cells to divide and grow, eventually leading to their death.

Chemotherapy can be effective at shrinking tumors and slowing the progression of advanced thyroid cancer, but it can also have side effects. The severity of these side effects varies according to the drugs used and the individual's overall health. Fatigue, nausea, hair loss, decreased appetite, and increased susceptibility to infections are common side effects of chemotherapy therapy. It is important to note, however, that not all individuals may have these side effects, and they can often be managed with support care measures.

Targeted Therapy

Targeted therapy is a relatively recent approach to treating cancer that focuses on specific molecular targets within cancer cells. Unlike chemotherapy, which affects both diseased and healthy cells, targeted therapy tries to attack cancer cells selectively while causing minimal damage to healthy cells. Precision targeting is done through the use of drugs that disrupt specific molecules or processes involved in cancer growth and progression.

Target therapy is primarily utilized in the treatment of thyroid cancer in advanced cases that are not responsive to other treatments or have spread to distant sites. The vascular endothelial growth factor receptor (VEGFR) is the most common molecular target in thyroid cancer, and it plays a role in stimulating the growth of blood vessels that give nutrients to tumors. Sorafenib and lenvatinib, two VEGFR inhibitors, have demonstrated encouraging effects in slowing the progression of advanced thyroid cancer.

In the form of pills or capsules, targeted therapy is often taken orally. The treatment is normally given once a day, and the duration of therapy varies based on the individual's response and tolerance to the medications. Regular monitoring and follow-up visits with the health care team are essential to assess the effectiveness of targeted therapy and manage any potential side effects.

Target therapy can be effective in suppressing the growth of advanced thyroid cancer, but it can also have side effects. These fat side effects can vary based on the specific medicine used, but they may include fatigue, high blood pressure, diarrhea, skin rash, and hand-foot syndrome. As there may be strategies to manage or mitigate these symptoms, it is important for individuals receiving targeted therapy to discuss any side effects with their healthcare team.

Finally, chemotherapy and targeted therapy are further thyroid cancer treatment options, particularly in advanced or metastatic cases. While chemotherapy is not commonly used as a first-line treatment for advanced thyroid cancer, it can be effective in reducing tumors and slowing the progression of the disease.

Targeted therapy, on the other hand, focuses on specific molecular targets within cancer cells and tries to kill cancer cells selectively while causing little damage to normal cells. Both treatment approaches have their own set of potential side effects, which are frequently managed with supportive care measures. Individuals need to review these treatment options with their healthcare team to determine the best course of action based on their specific condition.

Chapter 3

Recovery and Rehabilitation

Post-Surgery Recovery

It is important to focus on your post-surgery recovery after having surgery to treat thyroid cancer. This time is crucial for healing and recovering strength. In this section, we will outline what to expect during the recovery process and provide you with a few tips to help you successfully navigate this phase.

The Initial Recovery Period

You will be transferred to a recovery room immediately after surgery, where medical personnel will constantly monitor your vital signs. In the neck area, you may experience some discomfort, pain, or swelling, which is normal. Your healthcare team will provide you with pain medication to help you manage any discomfort.

It is common to have a drain in place during the early recovery period to remove any excess fluid or blood from the surgery site. Your healthcare team will explain how to care for the drain and when it can be removed.

A bandage or dressing may also be applied to the incision site. To prevent infection, it is important to keep the region clean and dry. Your healthcare team will provide you with advice on how to care for the incision site and when it is safe to remove the dressing.

Managing Pain and Discomfort

While discomfort and pain are normal after surgery, there are numerous strategies you can use to effectively manage them:

- **Take your pain medication exactly as prescribed:** Your healthcare team will provide you with pain medication to help you manage your discomfort. It is important to take the medication exactly as directed and not wait until the pain gets severe.

- **Apply ice packs to the surgical site:** Applying ice packs to the surgical site might help reduce swelling and provide relief. To avoid frostbite, cover the ice pack with a cloth or towel before applying it to your skin.

- **Practice relaxation techniques:** Deep breathing exercises, meditation, and guided imagery can help you relax and manage any pain or discomfort you may be experiencing.

- **Maintain a comfortable sleeping posture:** Finding a comfortable sleeping position after surgery might be challenging. Pillows to support your neck and head might help relieve discomfort and promote better sleep.

Resuming Activities

After surgery, it is important to resume normal activities gradually. But it's essential to listen to your body and avoid overexerting yourself. Following are some guidelines to follow:

- **Rest and take it easy:** Your body requires time to heal, so make sure to get plenty of rest. If necessary, take brief naps throughout the day and avoid vigorous activities.
- **Increase your physical activity gradually:** Begin with light activities like short walks and progressively increase the duration and intensity as you feel comfortable. Before beginning any workout program, consult with your healthcare team.
- **Avoid heavy lifting**: Avoid lifting heavy objects for at least a few weeks after surgery to avoid strain on your neck and incision site.
- **Follow dietary recommendations:** During your recovery, your healthcare team may provide specific dietary guidelines. To support healing and overall well-being, it is important to follow these recommendations.

Following-up Care and Monitoring

You will have regular follow-up appointments with your healthcare team during your post-surgery recovery. These meetings are essential for monitoring your progress and addressing any uncertainties or challenges that may occur.

Your healthcare team will most likely run blood tests to monitor your thyroid hormone levels and, if required, adjust your medication. They may also request imaging tests, such as ultrasound or radioactive iodine scans, to look for any residual cancer cells or symptoms of recurrence.

It is essential to attend all scheduled follow-up appointments and report any symptoms or health concerns you may have to your healthcare team. They are there to support you and ensure that your recovery is progressing as planned.

Emotional Support

It can be emotionally challenging to recover from thyroid cancer surgery. It is normal to experience several kinds of emotions, including anxiety, fear, and sadness. During this time, seeking emotional support from loved ones, support groups, or mental health specialists might be beneficial.

Consider joining a support group for thyroid cancer patients or connecting with other survivors who can provide direction and understanding. Additionally, engaging in self-care activities such as journaling, hobbies, or seeking therapy can help you navigate the emotional parts of your recovery.

Remember that everyone's recovery journey is different, and it's important to be patient and kind to yourself during this time. You may successfully navigate the post-surgery recovery phase and go forward on your path to flourishing after thyroid cancer with adequate care, support, and a positive outlook.

Managing Thyroid Hormone Levels

One of the most essential parts of your recovery and long-term management after undergoing thyroid cancer treatment is ensuring that your thyroid hormone levels are properly managed. The thyroid gland plays a crucial role in regulating various bodily functions, and maintaining the proper balance of thyroid hormones is crucial for your overall health and well-being.

The Importance of Thyroid Hormones

Thyroid hormones, primarily thyroxine (T4) and triiodothyronine (T3) regulate metabolism, growth, and development in the body. These hormones have an impact on practically every organ and tissue in the body, including the heart, brain, muscles, and digestive system. They help regulate the body's temperature, heart rate, energy levels, and even mood.

The thyroid gland may be partially or entirely removed in individuals who have undergone treatment for thyroid cancer, or its function may have been affected due to other treatment approaches. As a result, the body may be unable to create enough thyroid hormones on its own. Hypothyroidism is the term used to describe this condition.

Monitoring Thyroid Hormone Levels

Regular monitoring is essential to ensure that your thyroid hormone levels are correctly managed. Thyroid-stimulating hormone (TSH), T4, and T3 levels in your body will be measured by blood tests performed by your healthcare team. The pituitary gland produces TSH, which encourages the thyroid gland to create thyroid hormones. TSH levels that are too high indicate that your body is not making enough thyroid hormones, and medication adjustments may be required.

The goal of thyroid hormone replacement therapy is to maintain normal TSH levels, typically between 0.4 and 4.0 milliunits per liter (mU/L). Based on your specific circumstances, your healthcare professional will work closely with you to determine the proper dosage of thyroid hormone replacement medication. To ensure that your hormone levels are correctly managed, it is important to follow their instructions and attend regular follow-up sessions.

Thyroid Hormone Replacement Medication

Levothyroxine, a synthetic form of T4, is the most common form of thyroid hormone replacement medication. Levothyroxine is taken orally and is designed to mirror the body's natural thyroid hormone production. It is normally taken once a day on an empty stomach, ideally in the morning.

To maintain stable hormone levels, it is important to take your medication consistently and at the same time every day. Other medications or supplements that may interfere with levothyroxine absorption, such as calcium or iron supplements, should be avoided within a few hours of taking your thyroid hormone medication.

Your healthcare provider will prescribe an initial dosage of levothyroxine based on your body weight and the severity of your hypothyroidism. They may adjust the dosage over time based on your blood test results and any symptoms you are experiencing. It is crucial to communicate any changes in your health or overall well-being to your age care team, since this may indicate the need for a dosage adjustment.

Potential Side Effects and Interactions

Some individuals may experience side effects from thyroid hormone replacement medication, even though it is generally well tolerated. Headaches, fatigue, weight changes, hair loss, and bowel changes are some of the symptoms. If you experience any persistent or troublesome side effects, it is important to address them with your healthcare practitioner.

Certain medications and supplements can interfere with the absorption or effectiveness of thyroid hormone replacement medications. To avoid potential interactions, it is important to inform your healthcare practitioner about all medications, supplements, and herbal remedies you are taking. They can provide instructions on how to manage these interactions and, if necessary, adjust your medication.

Lifestyle Factors and Thyroid Hormone Levels

Aside from medication, several lifestyle factors can have an impact on your thyroid hormone levels. To support healthy thyroid function, it is important to maintain a healthy lifestyle. This includes the following:

- **Nutrition:** Eating a well-balanced diet rich in iodine-rich foods, including seafood, dairy products, and iodized salt, can help support thyroid health. Also important for thyroid health is ensuring appropriate selenium, zinc, and vitamin D intake.
- **Exercise:** Physical activity regularly can help improve thyroid function and metabolism. Walking, jogging, cycling, and weight training are all good activities. However, it is important to consult with your healthcare provider before beginning any new fitness plan.

- **Stress Management:** Chronic stress has been shown to impair thyroid function. Stress management practices such as meditation, deep breathing exercises, yoga, or engaging in hobbies can help reduce stress levels and support thyroid health.
- **Avoiding Smoking and Excessive Alcohol Consumption:** Thyroid function and hormone metabolism can be interfered with by smoking and excessive alcohol consumption. Quitting smoking and minimizing alcohol intake can improve thyroid health.

You may support your recovery and overall well-being after thyroid cancer treatment by adopting these lifestyle factors into your daily routine and working together with your healthcare team to manage your thyroid hormone levels. Remember to keep your follow-up appointments, communicate any changes in symptoms or well-being, and take your medication as directed to ensure that your thyroid hormone levels are managed optimally.

Dealing with Side Effects of Treatment

We have discussed the many treatment options for thyroid cancer in previous sections, including surgery, radioactive iodine therapy, external beam radiation therapy, and chemotherapy. While these treatments are essential in combating cancer and preventing its spread, they can also have side effects that affect your quality of life during and after treatment.

In this part, we'll look at some of the most common side effects of thyroid cancer treatment and provide strategies to help you manage and cope with them effectively. It's important to remember that everyone's experience with essential health care may differ, and it's important to consult with your essential health team for tailored advice and support.

Recognizing Common Side Effects

Fatigue is a common side effect reported by many cancer patients, including those undergoing thyroid cancer treatment. It can be caused by a combination of factors, such as the physical and emotional stress of the diagnosis and treatment, changes in hormone levels, and the body's healing process. To manage fatigue, it is important to prioritize rest and sleep, conserve energy by delegating duties, and engage in light exercise or relaxing activities such as yoga or meditation.

- **Hair Loss:** Some thyroid cancer treatments, such as chemotherapy, might result in temporary hair loss. This can be stressful for many individuals, as hair loss can have an impact on self-esteem and body image. Consider using wigs, scarves, or hats to conceal your hair loss, or embrace your new look with confidence.

Keep in mind that hair loss is usually transient, and your hair will most likely regrow after treatment.

- **Nausea and Vomiting:** Certain treatments, such as chemotherapy, can cause nausea and vomiting. It is important to communicate any nausea symptoms to your healthcare team, as they can prescribe medications or recommend dietary changes to reduce these symptoms. Eating small, frequent meals, avoiding strong odors or triggers, and staying hydrated can also help with nausea management.

- **Changes in Appetite and Taste:** Thyroid cancer treatment can occasionally alter your appetite and taste preferences. You may experience a loss of appetite or taste changes. To support your body's healing process, it is important to maintain healthy nourishment throughout this time. Consider eating small, regular meals that are high in nutrients and delicious. Experiment with various flavors and textures to find foods that are both delicious and simple to eat.

- **Dry Mouth and Difficulty Swallowing:** After receiving treatment for thyroid cancer, some individuals may experience dry mouth and difficulty swallowing. This could be due to radiation therapy's effects on the salivary glands and throat. To relieve dry mouth, drink plenty of water, use sugar-free candies or gum to increase saliva production, and avoid dry or spicy foods. If swallowing becomes challenging, consult your healthcare team for advice and possible interventions.

- **Skin Changes:** Skin changes in the treated area may occur from time to time as a result of radiation therapy. These symptoms may include redness, dryness, itching, or peeling. It's important to keep the skin clean and moisturized, avoid direct sunlight exposure, and wear loose-fitting clothing to avoid friction and irritation. Consult your healthcare team for recommended skin care products and strategies to effectively manage these skin changes.

- **Emotional and Psychological Effects:** Coping with a cancer diagnosis and undergoing treatment can have a significant impact on your emotional and psychological well-being. Fear, anxiety, sadness, and rage are all normal feelings to experience. To help you navigate these feelings, consider seeking help from a therapist, counselor, or support group. Participating in activities that bring you joy, practicing self-care, and maintaining open communication with your loved ones can all contribute to your emotional well-being.

Seeking Support and Guidance

Managing the side effects of thyroid cancer treatment can be challenging, but you don't have to go through it alone. It is important to communicate freely with your healthcare team about any side effects you are experiencing. They can provide assistance, prescribe medications if necessary, and provide coping strategies to help you manage effectively.

Additionally, try reaching out to thyroid cancer support groups or organizations. Connecting with others who have had similar experiences can provide useful insights, emotional support, and practical ideas for dealing with side effects.

As you navigate through the side effects of treatment, remember to be patient with yourself. Each person's journey is unique, and finding the strategies that work best for you may take some time. You may effectively manage the side effects of thyroid cancer treatment and continue on your path to recovery and thriving with the correct support, self-care, and a positive outlook.

Nutrition and Exercise for Recovery

In this section will discuss the importance of nutrition and exercise in the recovery of thyroid cancer. Both nutrition and exercise play crucial roles in helping the body's healing process, boosting energy levels, and improving overall well-being.

The Role of Nutrition in Recovery

For individuals recovering from thyroid cancer, proper nutrition is essential. A healthy diet can help support the immune system, promote healing, and provide the nutrients the body requires to function properly. Here are some crucial nutritional concerns for recovery:

- **Adequate Caloric Intake:** It is important to consume enough calories to meet the body's energy needs during recovery. This may involve modestly boosting calorie intake to support recovery and prevent weight loss. Working with a licensed dietitian can help you determine the best calorie intake for your needs.

- **Nutrient-Dense Foods:** Choose nutrient-dense foods that provide a variety of vitamins, minerals, and antioxidants. Incorporate plenty of fruits and vegetables, whole grains, lean proteins, and healthy fats into your diet. These foods can help support the immune system and speed up the healing process.

- **Protein-Rich Foods:** Protein is crucial for tissue repair and recovery. Include lean protein sources in your meals, such as fowl, fish, beans, lentils, tofu, and Greek yogurt. Aim for a balanced protein intake throughout the day.

- **Hydration:** Staying hydrated is important for overall health and recovery. Drink enough water throughout the day to support digestion, circulation, and detoxification. Caffeine and alcohol, in excess, can dehydrate the body.

- **Supplements:** In some cases, individuals recovering from thyroid cancer may require specific supplements to treat vitamin shortages. Work with your healthcare team to determine whether supplements are required and to ensure that they do not interfere with your treatment.

- **Manage Side Effects:** Some thyroid cancer treatments, such as radioactive iodine therapy, may cause transient taste changes or difficulties swallowing. Work with a certified dietitian to discover strategies to manage these side effects and ensure proper nutrition if you experience any of these side effects.

The Importance of Exercise in Recovery

For individuals with thyroid cancer, exercise is an important component of the recovery process. Regular physical activity can provide a variety of advantages, including:

- **Improved Energy Levels:** Regular exercise can help overcome fatigue and boost overall energy levels. Begin with low-impact activities like walking, swimming, or cycling, then gradually increase the intensity as tolerated.

- **Enhanced Mood and Mental Well-Being:** Exercise has been shown to release endorphins, which can improve mood and reduce feelings of anxiety and depression. It can also serve as a positive distraction and help individuals deal with the emotional challenges associated with a cancer diagnosis.

- **Maintained Muscle Strength and Bone Health:** Certain treatments for thyroid cancer, such as surgery and radioactive iodine therapy, may lead to muscle weakness and bone loss. Exercise, including strength training and weight-bearing activities, can help to maintain muscle strength and bone density.

- **Improved Cardiovascular Health:** Engaging in aerobic exercise can improve cardiovascular health, increase endurance, and enhance overall fitness. Consult your healthcare team to determine the best amount of intensity and duration for your exercise routine.

- **Weight Management:** Regular exercise, combined with a well-balanced diet, can help with weight management both during and after treatment. Maintaining a healthy weight is important for overall health as well as reducing the risk of cancer recurrence.

- **Social Support:** Participating in group exercise classes or engaging in physical activities with friends and family during the recovery process can provide social support and a sense of community.

Tips for Incorporating Nutrition and Exercise into Recovery

Here are some helpful hints for incorporating nutrition and exercise into your thyroid cancer recovery:

- **Consult a Registered Dietitian:** Consult with a registered dietitian who specializes in cancer nutrition to develop a personalized meal plan that suits your specific needs and interests.

- **Start Slowly with Exercise:** Begin with low-impact exercises and gradually increase intensity and duration as your energy levels and fitness improve. Listen to your body and take breaks as needed.

- **Stay Consistent:** Aim for regular exercise and make it a part of your daily routine. The key to obtaining the advantages of physical activity is consistency.

- **Seek Professional Guidance:** If you are unclear about the appropriate exercises or have concerns about your physical skills, consult with a physical therapist or exercise specialist who can walk you through a safe and effective exercise regimen.

- **Stay Positive:** Thyroid cancer recovery can be challenging, but maintaining a positive attitude and concentrating on self-care can make a major difference. Surround yourself with a strong support network of family, friends, and healthcare experts.

Remember that each person's recovery journey is unique. It is important to work closely with your healthcare team to develop a personalized nutrition and exercise plan that meets your specific health needs and medical conditions. You may support your body's healing process, enhance your overall well-being, and thrive after thyroid cancer by prioritizing nutrition and exercise.

Emotional and Psychological Support

Receiving a thyroid cancer diagnosis can be a disruptive and emotionally challenging experience. Along with the physical components of treatment and recovery, it is crucial to address the emotional and psychological side of the disease. Emotional support plays an important role in helping individuals navigate the various stages of thyroid cancer, from diagnosis to treatment and beyond. This section will discuss the importance of emotional and psychological support as well as provide strategies for dealing with the emotional challenges that come with thyroid cancer.

The Emotional Impact of Thyroid Cancer

For both individuals and their loved ones, Thyroid Cancer can have a significant emotional impact. Fear, anxiety, sadness, anger, and confusion are all emotions that might be triggered by a diagnosis. It is normal to experience these emotions and to feel overwhelmed by the uncertainty that comes with a cancer diagnosis. Furthermore, physical changes caused by treatment, such as weight fluctuations, hair loss, and changes in appearance, might contribute to emotional distress.

Seeking Support

During this challenging time, it is essential to acknowledge the importance of seeking support. Having a solid support network can provide you with comfort, understanding, and encouragement during your thyroid cancer journey. Seeking emotional and psychological support might take the following routes:

1. Relatives and friends

Seek emotional support from your loved ones. Allow them to be there for you by sharing your feelings and concerns with them. Their presence and understanding can provide a sense of security and comfort.

2. Support Organizations

Joining a support group designed exclusively for thyroid cancer patients can be quite beneficial. Connecting with others who are experiencing or have experienced similar situations can provide a sense of belonging and understanding. Support groups provide a safe area for people to express their emotions, share knowledge, and learn from the experiences of others.

3. Professionals in Mental Health

Consider seeking the assistance of a mental health expert who specializes in difficulties related to cancer, such as a therapist or counselor. They can provide guidance and support in dealing with the emotional challenges that come with thyroid cancer. Therapy can help individuals develop their coping strategies, improve their communication skills, and address any underlying mental health concerns.

4. Online Communities

Participating in thyroid cancer-specific online communities and forums can be a helpful source of support. Individuals can connect with others across the world, share experiences, ask questions, and receive support and guidance from a broad group of people who understand the challenges of living with thyroid cancer through these platforms.

Coping Strategies

Implementing coping strategies can help individuals manage the emotional effects of thyroid cancer, in addition to seeking support. Consider the following strategies:

1. Express Your Emotions

Allow yourself to openly and honestly express your emotions. Finding healthy ways to express your feelings, whether through writing, talking to a trusted friend, or engaging in creative outlets such as art or music, can provide a sense of comfort and release.

2. Practice Self-Care

Make self-care activities that promote relaxation and well-being a priority. Engage in activities that bring you delight, such as reading, listening to music, practicing mindfulness or meditation, taking walks in nature, or engaging in hobbies. Taking care of your physical and emotional well-being is crucial during this time.

3. Educate Yourself

Knowledge is empowering. Learn about thyroid cancer, options for treatment, and the recovery process. Understanding the disease and how it is managed can help reduce anxiety and provide a sense of control.

4. Communicate with Your Healthcare Team

Keep an open and honest line of communication with your healthcare team. Discuss any concerns or fears you may have, as well as any questions you may have concerning your treatment plan and prognosis. Being informed and participating in your care can help reduce anxiety and increase confidence in the treatment process.

5. Practice Stress Management Techniques

Explore stress management methods that work for you. Deep breathing exercises, gradual muscle relaxation, yoga, or engaging in activities that promote relaxation and stress reduction may be included. Finding healthy strategies to manage stress can improve your well-being and help you deal with the emotional challenges of thyroid cancer.

Emotional and psychological support are essential components of the thyroid cancer journey. Seeking support from loved ones, participating in support groups, and engaging with mental health specialists can provide the necessary direction and understanding during this challenging time.

Implementing coping strategies and engaging in self-care can help individuals navigate the emotional burden of thyroid cancer and promote overall well-being. Remember that you are not alone and that there is support available to help you through every stage of your thyroid cancer journey.

Chapter 4

Living with Thyroid Cancer

Long-Term Monitoring and Follow-Up

It is crucial to establish a long-term follow-up and monitoring strategy after completing your initial thyroid cancer treatment. Regular follow-up visits and monitoring tests are essential to ensure that your cancer is under control and to detect any potential recurrence or metastasis at an early stage. In this section, we will discuss the importance of long-term follow-up, the recommended monitoring tests, and what to expect during these visits.

The Importance of Long-Term Follow-Up

Thyroid cancer has a high rate of survival, especially when detected and treated early. It is important to note, however, that thyroid cancer can reappear even years after treatment. Regular follow-up visits enable your healthcare team to monitor your progress, detect signs of recurrence or metastasis, and provide appropriate interventions as needed. These visits also provide an opportunity to discuss any concerns or questions you may have about your health and well-being.

Recommended Monitoring Tests

Your healthcare provider will recommend particular monitoring tests during your long-term follow-up based on the type and stage of your thyroid cancer as well as the treatment you received. Some popular tests that may be included in your monitoring plan are as follows:

- **Thyroid Hormone Levels:** It is crucial to monitor your thyroid hormone levels, including TSH, T3, and T4, to ensure that your thyroid function is steady. If necessary, your healthcare team will change your thyroid hormone replacement medicine.

- **Neck Ultrasound:** A non-invasive imaging procedure that employs sound waves to obtain detailed images of the thyroid gland and surrounding structures is a neck ultrasound. It aids in the detection of any changes in thyroid gland size or appearance, as well as the presence of any worrisome nodules.

- **Blood Test for Thyroglobulin (Tg):** Thyroglobulin is a protein generated by both normal and malignant thyroid cells. A blood test to evaluate thyroglobulin levels is frequently used as a tumor marker for thyroid cancer monitoring. The presence of residual or recurring cancer may be indicated by elevated thyroglobulin levels.

- **Radioactive Iodine (RAI) Whole Body Scan:** If you received radioactive iodine therapy as part of your treatment, your healthcare team may recommend periodic whole-body scans to detect any remaining or recurrent thyroid cancer cells. A small amount of radioactive iodine is administered during this scan, which is taken up by thyroid cells and detected by a particular camera.

- **Chest X-ray:** A chest X-ray may be performed to check for the presence of any lung metastases or other abnormalities in the chest area.

- **Computed Tomography (CT) Scan:** A CT scan uses X-rays and computer technology to create detailed cross-sectional images of the body. To check for the presence of cancer or metastasis, it may be necessary to evaluate the neck, chest, or other locations.

- **Positron Emission Tomography (PET) Scan:** A PET scan is a nuclear medicine imaging test that uses a radioactive tracer to detect areas of increased metabolic activity in the body. It can aid in the detection of cancer recurrence or metastasis in several organs.

Follow-Up Visits

You will have the opportunity to discuss any concerns or symptoms you may be experiencing with your healthcare team at your follow-up visits. They will perform a physical examination, evaluate your medical history, and order any monitoring tests that are required. The number of follow-up visits you need may vary based on the type and stage of your thyroid cancer, as well as the treatment you received. In general, follow-up visits should be scheduled every 6 to 12 months for the first few years following treatment, and then less frequently as time passes.

Your healthcare team will assess your overall health, monitor your thyroid hormone levels, and evaluate the findings of any imaging or blood tests during these visits. They will discuss the findings with you and provide recommendations for any necessary interventions or changes to your treatment plan. These visits also provide you with the opportunity to ask questions, get emotional support, and discuss any lifestyle changes or concerns you may have.

Self-Awareness and Self-Care

It is important to be proactive in self-monitoring and self-care in addition to regular follow-up visits. Any changes in your body, such as the appearance of new tumors or nodules, trouble swallowing or breathing, unexplained weight loss or gain, or persistent exhaustion, should be noted. If you detect any troubling symptoms, please contact your healthcare team as soon as possible.

Maintaining a healthy lifestyle is also crucial for long-term well-being. Eat a well-balanced diet, exercise regularly, and avoid cigarettes and excessive alcohol usage. Take your medications as prescribed and attend all specified follow-up visits and monitoring tests. You can improve your chances of long-term success in thyroid cancer management by actively participating in your care.

Finally, establishing a long-term follow-up and monitoring strategy is essential for those who have undergone thyroid cancer treatment. Regular follow-up visits and monitoring tests enable healthcare providers to detect early signs of recurrence or metastasis and provide necessary interventions. You can regain control of your health and thrive after thyroid cancer by actively participating in your follow-up care and maintaining a healthy lifestyle.

Managing Recurrence and Metastasis

Thyroid cancer recurrence and metastasis can be a challenging and frustrating experience for people who have already received treatment. The return of cancer cells in the thyroid or nearby lymph nodes after initial treatment is referred to as recurrence, whereas metastasis occurs when cancer cells spread to other organs or tissues in the body.

Although the prospect of cancer reoccurring or spreading can be frightening, it is important to remember that there are techniques and treatments available to help manage and treat these circumstances.

Recognizing Recurrence and Metastasis

Depending on the type and stage of thyroid cancer, recurrence, and metastasis can occur in a variety of ways. A local recurrence in the thyroid bed or nearby lymph nodes may result from cancer cells that were left behind after surgery or treatment in some cases. In some cases, cancer cells may have spread to distant organs such as the lungs, bones, or liver, resulting in metastasis.

It is crucial for individuals who have undergone thyroid cancer treatment to be cautious and attend regular follow-up checkups and monitoring. This enables healthcare providers to detect early signs of recurrence or metastasis and come up with a suitable treatment plan.

Diagnostic Tests for Recurrence and Metastasis

Various diagnostic tests may be performed to evaluate the extent and location of the cancer when there is suspicion of recurrence or metastasis. These tests may involve the following:

- **Imaging tests:** Imaging techniques such as ultrasound, computed tomography (CT) scans, magnetic resonance imaging (MRI), or positron emission tomography (PET) scans can help identify the presence and location of cancer cells in the body.

- **Blood tests:** Blood tests, including thyroglobulin and calcitonin levels, can be used to monitor tumor markers. Elevated levels of these markers can indicate the presence of recurrent or metastatic thyroid cancer.

- **Biopsy:** If a suspicious area is identified through imaging tests, a biopsy may be performed to obtain a tissue sample for further analysis. This can assist in confirming the presence of cancer cells and characterizing them.

Treatment Options for Recurrence and Metastasis

The type of cancer, the extent of the disease, and the individual's overall health all have a role in the treatment strategy for thyroid cancer recurrence and metastasis. Among the treatment alternatives that may be considered are:

- **Surgery:** In cases where the recurrence or metastasis is confined, surgical intervention to remove the damaged thyroid tissue or metastatic lesions may be advised. This can help relieve symptoms and possibly remove cancer cells.

- **Radioactive iodine therapy:** Radioactive iodine therapy, also known as I-131 therapy, may be used to target and destroy remaining thyroid tissue or cancer cells that have absorbed iodine. This treatment is especially helpful for specific kinds of thyroid cancer that can still absorb iodine.

- **External beam radiation therapy:** External beam radiation therapy involves the use of high-energy

X-rays or protons to target and destroy cancer cells. This treatment may be utilized to manage recurrent or metastatic thyroid cancer that is unable to be eliminated surgically.

- **Systemic therapies:** Systemic therapies, such as chemotherapy or targeted therapy, may be considered for advanced cases of recurrent or metastatic thyroid cancer. These medicines work by specifically targeting substances or pathways involved in cancer growth and spread.

- **Clinical trials:** Participation in clinical trials may be an option for individuals with recurrent or metastatic thyroid cancer. Clinical trials allow patients to have access to novel treatments and therapies that are not yet broadly available.

Supportive Care and Emotional Well-Being

Managing recurrence and metastasis can be physically and emotionally challenging. Individuals need to seek support from healthcare experts, support groups, and loved ones during this challenging time. Measures of support may include:

- **Pain management:** If recurrent or metastatic thyroid cancer causes pain or discomfort, various pain management techniques and medications can be utilized to alleviate symptoms and improve quality of life.

- **Symptom management:** Individuals with cancer may experience a variety of symptoms, such as fatigue, trouble swallowing, or shortness of breath, depending on the location and extent of the cancer. Supportive treatment can aid in the management of these symptoms and enhance overall comfort.

- **Psychological support:** Dealing with a thyroid cancer recurrence or metastasis can be emotionally draining. Counseling or joining support groups can provide individuals with a secure area to express their thoughts, discuss their experiences, and get emotional support.

- **Healthy lifestyle practices:** Maintaining a healthy lifestyle through regular exercise, proper nutrition, and stress management techniques can help individuals cope with the challenges of managing recurrent or metastatic thyroid cancer.

Prognosis and Hope

While dealing with recurrence and metastasis might be overwhelming, it is important to remember that there is still hope. The prognosis for individuals with recurrent or metastatic thyroid cancer has considerably improved due to advancements in medical research and treatment options. Individuals can negotiate the challenges of managing thyroid cancer health recurrence and metastasis with perseverance and hope by working closely with healthcare experts, remaining updated about the latest treatment options, and maintaining a positive mentality.

Palliative and Supportive Care

Supportive and palliative care are crucial in the overall management of thyroid cancer. While supportive care focuses on assisting and comforting patients during their treatment journey, palliative care aims to improve the quality of life for individuals suffering from advanced or incurable thyroid cancer. This section will discuss the importance of supportive care and palliative care in thyroid cancer, as well as the numerous strategies and resources accessible to patients.

The Importance of Supportive Care

Supportive care is an essential component of thyroid cancer treatment as it addresses the physical, emotional, and practical needs of patients. By treating symptoms, decreasing treatment side effects, and improving their ability to cope with the challenges of the disease, it aims to enhance the overall well-being of individuals. Supportive care can be provided by a multidisciplinary team of healthcare experts, which may include oncologists, nurses, social workers, psychologists, and dietitians.

One of the key purposes of supportive care is to manage thyroid cancer treatment side effects. Surgery, radioactive iodine therapy, external beam radiation therapy, and chemotherapy can all cause pain, exhaustion, nausea, hair loss, and appetite changes. Pain management strategies, anti-nausea drugs, and dietary advice are examples of supportive care interventions that can help these symptoms and improve the patient's overall comfort.

Supportive care also focuses on the emotional and psychological effects of thyroid cancer. An emotionally upsetting cancer diagnosis can cause anxiety, despair, and terror. Counseling, support groups, and other psychological interventions can be provided by supportive care providers to assist patients and their families in navigating the emotional challenges associated with the disease. They can also help with practical concerns, such as financial and logistical issues related to treatment.

Palliative Care for Advanced Thyroid Cancer

Palliative care is a type of supportive care that is especially important for individuals with advanced or incurable thyroid cancer. It focuses on improving patients' quality of life by controlling symptoms, offering emotional support, and addressing spiritual and existential concerns. Palliative care can begin at any stage of the disease and can be provided in conjunction with curative therapy.

Palliative care aims to reduce symptoms and enhance the patient's comfort. Medication may be used to manage pain, nausea, shortness of breath, and other uncomfortable symptoms. Palliative care providers collaborate with patients and their families to create tailored care plans that suit their specific needs and preferences.

Palliative care stresses emotional support in addition to symptom control. The emotional and existential challenges that patients with advanced thyroid cancer encounter are enormous. Palliative care experts can provide counseling, spiritual advice, and aid with advance care planning to assist patients in navigating these tough talks and decisions.

It is important to understand that palliative care is not the same as end-of-life care. While palliative care addresses end-of-life concerns, its major focus is on improving the patient's quality of life throughout their illness. Palliative care can be provided in conjunction with curative therapy and can continue even if the disease advances.

Resources for Supportive Care and Palliative Care

There are various resources accessible to individuals receiving supportive and palliative care for thyroid cancer. These resources can provide patients and their families with essential information, counseling, and support. Among the most important resources are:

- Joining a support group might provide an opportunity to connect with others who are going through similar circumstances. These groups provide a secure area for individuals to share their emotions, exchange practical advice, and seek support from those who understand the challenges of living with thyroid cancer.

- Palliative care teams are made up of healthcare experts who are skilled at managing symptoms, offering emotional support, and addressing spiritual and existential concerns. They collaborate closely with patients and their families to create personalized care plans and ensure that their requirements are satisfied throughout the illness.

- Hospice care is a type of palliative care that focuses on providing comfort and support to individuals with a life-limiting condition. Hospice care can be provided in a variety of venues, such as hospitals, nursing homes, and patients' homes. During the terminal stages of the disease, it aims to enhance the quality of life for patients and their families.

- There are various respectable websites and online forums dedicated to offering information and support to individuals suffering from thyroid cancer. These resources provide patients with educational materials, discussion forums, and access to professional counsel, helping them to stay educated and connected throughout their treatment experience.

- Social workers and patient navigators can help patients and their families get access to supportive care and palliative care services. They can advise on available resources, assist with financial and logistical concerns, and provide emotional support during the treatment process.

Finally, supportive and palliative care are essential components of thyroid cancer management. By treating symptoms, addressing emotional and practical needs, and improving quality of life, they seek to enhance patients' overall well-being. Individuals with thyroid cancer can obtain the support and comfort they need to navigate their treatment journey with resilience and comfort by utilizing the available resources and collaborating closely with healthcare providers.

Keeping a Healthy Lifestyle

For individuals with thyroid cancer, maintaining a healthy lifestyle is crucial. Adopting healthy behaviors can not only support recovery but also improve overall well-being and reduce the risk of recurrence. In this section, we'll look at many components of living a healthy lifestyle, such as food, exercise, stress management, and avoiding dangerous substances.

Diet

A well-balanced and healthy diet is essential for immune system support and overall health. While no single diet may cure thyroid cancer, several dietary choices can aid in recovery and reduce the risk of complications. Here are some important considerations:

- **Nutrient-dense foods:** Eat a variety of fruits and vegetables, whole grains, lean proteins, and healthy fats. These foods provide the body with essential vitamins, minerals, and antioxidants that support the healing process.

- **Iodine intake:** Iodine is essential for thyroid function, but excessive iodine intake can be harmful, especially for individuals with certain types of thyroid cancer. Consult your healthcare professional to discover the recommended level of iodine intake for your unique condition.

- **Reduce your intake of processed foods:** Processed foods can contain high levels of harmful fats, sodium, and additives. Reduce your consumption of processed foods and replace them with fresh, natural foods wherever possible.

- **Hydration:** Drink plenty of water throughout the day to stay hydrated. Proper hydration helps maintain healthy physiological processes and supports overall health.

- **Moderate caffeine and alcohol consumption:** While moderate consumption of caffeine and alcohol is generally acceptable, excessive intake can negatively impact your health. Limit your consumption of caffeinated beverages and alcohol, as they can disrupt your sleep patterns and overall well-being.

Physical Activity

Individuals with thyroid cancer should exercise regularly because it is beneficial to everyone. Exercise not only helps you maintain a healthy weight, but it also helps you improve your cardiovascular health, mood, and general quality of life. When incorporating exercise into your routine, keep the following things in mind:

- **Consult your healthcare provider:** Before starting any exercise program, consult with your healthcare provider to ensure it is safe and appropriate for your specific condition.

- **Begin slowly:** If you have been inactive for a long time or are recovering from surgery or treatment, begin with gentle exercises like walking or stretching. As your strength and stamina improve, gradually increase the intensity and duration of your workouts.

- **Select activities that you enjoy:** Take part in activities that you find enjoyable and long-lasting. Walking, swimming, cycling, yoga, and any other form of exercise that meets your interests and talents could all be included.

- **Strength training:** Incorporate strength training exercises into your routine to improve bone health and muscle strength. This can be accomplished with the use of weights, resistance bands, or bodyweight exercises.

- **Pay attention to your body:** Consider how your body feels during and after exercise. Modify your routine or consult with your healthcare practitioner if you develop pain, exhaustion, or other discomfort.

Stress Management

Stress management is essential for overall well-being and can be especially beneficial for individuals with thyroid cancer. Chronic stress can harm the immune system and impede recovery. Consider the following stress-management strategies:

- **Relaxation techniques:** Practice relaxation techniques such as deep breathing, meditation, or yoga to promote a sense of calm and reduce stress levels.

- **Engage in enjoyable activities:** Look for activities that will make you happy and help you relax. This could include activities such as hobbies, spending time in nature, listening to music, or engaging in creative endeavors.

- **Prioritize self-care:** Make self-care a priority by setting aside time for activities that promote relaxation and well-being. Taking baths, reading, journaling, or engaging in mindfulness techniques are examples of such activities.

- **Seek support:** Speak with friends, relatives, or support groups who can provide emotional support and understanding. Sharing your feelings and experiences with people who have had similar challenges can be quite beneficial.

Staying Away from Harmful Substances

Certain substances can be harmful to your health and increase your risk of complications. To support your recovery and overall well-being, it is important to avoid or limit your exposure to these substances. Take a look at the following:

- **Tobacco:** Smoking and secondhand smoke exposure can increase the risk of a variety of health disorders, including cancer. If you smoke, seek support to quit and avoid secondhand smoke exposure.

- **Environmental toxins:** Minimize exposure to environmental toxins such as pesticides, chemicals, and pollutants. When feasible, use natural cleaning products, eat organic foods, and be careful of your environment.

- **Harmful Substances:** Reduce or avoid the consumption of substances that can harm your health, such as recreational drugs or excessive alcohol consumption.

Individuals with thyroid cancer can manage their health, reduce the risk of problems, and improve their overall well-being by adopting a healthy lifestyle that includes a balanced diet, frequent exercise, stress management, and avoiding dangerous substances. Before making any big changes to your lifestyle or starting a fresh exercise routine, consult with your healthcare practitioner.

Chapter 5

Thriving after Thyroid Cancer

Creating a Survivorship Plan

After completing treatment for thyroid cancer, it is important to create a survivorship plan to help you navigate the next phase of your journey. A survivorship plan is a personalized roadmap that outlines the necessary steps and strategies to ensure your long-term health and well-being.

This plan will address various aspects of your life, including physical, emotional, and practical considerations. By creating a survivorship plan, you can take control of your future and thrive after thyroid cancer.

Understanding the Purpose of a Survivorship Plan

A survivorship plan serves several purposes. Firstly, it provides a comprehensive summary of your diagnosis, treatment, and follow-up care. This information is crucial for you and your healthcare team to have a clear understanding of your medical history and the steps that have been taken to manage your thyroid cancer. Additionally, a survivorship plan helps you stay organized and informed about your ongoing healthcare needs.

Secondly, a survivorship plan outlines the recommended follow-up care and monitoring schedule. Regular check-ups and tests are essential to detect any potential recurrence or complications early on. By adhering to the follow-up plan outlined in your survivorship plan, you can ensure that you receive the necessary medical attention and support.

Lastly, a survivorship plan addresses the physical, emotional, and practical aspects of life after thyroid cancer. It guides managing potential long-term side effects, maintaining a healthy lifestyle, and seeking support when needed. By considering all these factors, a survivorship plan helps you transition from being a cancer patient to a cancer survivor.

Components of a Survivorship Plan

A comprehensive survivorship plan should include the following components:

1. Medical Summary

This section provides a detailed summary of your thyroid cancer diagnosis, including the type and stage of cancer, treatments received, and any complications or side effects experienced. It also includes a list of your healthcare providers and their contact information.

2. Follow-Up Care

This section outlines the recommended follow-up care and monitoring schedule. It includes information about the frequency of check-ups, blood tests, imaging studies, and other diagnostic procedures. It is important to adhere to this schedule to ensure early detection of any potential recurrence or complications.

3. Managing Long-Term Side Effects

Thyroid cancer treatment can sometimes result in long-term side effects, such as changes in thyroid hormone levels, fatigue, weight gain, or difficulty swallowing. This section provides strategies for managing these side effects and improving your quality of life. It may include recommendations for medication adjustments, dietary modifications, exercise routines, and other supportive therapies.

4. Healthy Lifestyle Recommendations

Maintaining a healthy lifestyle is crucial for your overall well-being after thyroid cancer. This section provides guidance on nutrition, exercise, and stress management techniques. It may include tips for adopting a balanced diet, engaging in regular physical activity, and practicing relaxation techniques such as meditation or yoga.

5. Emotional and Psychological Support

Dealing with a cancer diagnosis and treatment can take a toll on your emotional well-being. This section addresses the importance of seeking emotional support and provides resources for counseling, support groups, or online communities. It may also include strategies for coping with anxiety, fear of recurrence, or body image issues.

6. Financial and Practical Considerations

Thyroid cancer treatment can be costly, and it is important to address any financial concerns or practical challenges that may arise. This section provides information on insurance coverage, financial assistance programs, and resources for managing the practical aspects of life after cancer, such as employment, education, or childcare.

Implementing Your Survivorship Plan

Creating a survivorship plan is just the first step. It is important to actively implement the strategies and recommendations outlined in your plan. This involves scheduling and attending regular follow-up appointments, adhering to medication regimens, adopting a healthy lifestyle, and seeking support when needed.

Regular communication with your healthcare team is essential. Keep them informed about any changes in your health or concerns you may have. They can provide guidance, answer your questions, and make adjustments to your survivorship plan as needed.

Remember that your survivorship plan is a living document that can be updated and modified over time. As you progress in your recovery and gain a better understanding of your needs, you can make adjustments to your plan accordingly.

By creating and implementing a survivorship plan, you are taking an active role in your well-being and ensuring a brighter future after thyroid cancer. Embrace the opportunities for growth and continue to thrive as a cancer survivor.

Building a Support Network

Dealing with thyroid cancer can be a challenging and overwhelming experience. It is important to remember that you do not have to face it alone. Building a strong support network can provide you with the emotional, practical, and informational support you need throughout your journey. In this section, we will explore the importance of a support network and provide you with strategies to build and maintain one.

The Importance of a Support Network

A support network is a group of individuals who are there to offer you encouragement, understanding, and assistance during your thyroid cancer journey. They can include family members, friends, healthcare professionals, support groups, and online communities. Here are some reasons why building a support network is crucial:

- **Emotional Support:** Dealing with a cancer diagnosis can bring about a range of emotions, including fear, anxiety, and sadness. Having a support network allows you to express your feelings and receive empathy and understanding from others who have been through similar experiences.

- **Practical Support:** Treatment for thyroid cancer may involve various appointments, medications, and lifestyle adjustments. A support network can help you with practical tasks such as transportation to appointments, meal preparation, and childcare, easing the burden on you and your loved ones.

- **Information and Resources:** Your support network can provide you with valuable information about treatment options, side effects, and coping strategies. They can also connect you with resources such as reputable websites, books, and support groups that can further enhance your knowledge and understanding of thyroid cancer.

- **Motivation and Encouragement:** Having a support network can provide you with the motivation and encouragement you need to stay positive and focused on your recovery. They can celebrate your milestones, offer words of encouragement, and remind you of your strength and resilience.

Strategies for Building a Support Network

Building a support network may take time and effort, but the benefits are well worth it. Here are some strategies to help you build and maintain a strong support network:

1. **Communicate with your loved ones:** Start by reaching out to your family and close friends. Share your diagnosis, treatment plan, and any specific needs or concerns you may have. Open and honest communication is key to building a strong support network.

2. **Seek support groups:** Joining a support group specifically for thyroid cancer patients can be incredibly beneficial. These groups provide a safe space to share experiences, ask questions, and receive support from individuals who truly understand what you are going through. Ask your healthcare provider or search online for local or online support groups.

3. **Utilize online communities:** The internet offers a wealth of resources and online communities for individuals with thyroid cancer. Joining online forums, and social media groups, or participating in virtual support groups can connect you with others who can offer support and advice.

4. **Connect with healthcare professionals:** Your healthcare team can be an essential part of your support network. They can provide you with medical

information, answer your questions, and refer you to additional resources. Building a trusting relationship with your healthcare providers can make a significant difference in your journey.

5. **Consider professional counseling:** Dealing with a cancer diagnosis can be emotionally challenging. Seeking the help of a professional counselor or therapist can provide you with a safe space to process your emotions, develop coping strategies, and gain additional support.

6. **Engage in community activities:** Participating in community activities, such as cancer awareness events or fundraising walks, can connect you with other individuals who have been affected by cancer. These events provide an opportunity to meet new people, share experiences, and build connections.

7. **Lean on your faith or spirituality:** If you have a religious or spiritual practice, reaching out to your faith community can provide you with additional support and comfort during difficult times. Many religious organizations offer support groups or pastoral care services for individuals facing health challenges.

Maintaining Your Support Network

Building a support network is not a one-time task; it requires ongoing effort and maintenance. Here are some tips for maintaining your support network:

1. **Express gratitude:** Show appreciation to your support network by expressing gratitude for their presence and assistance. A simple thank-you can go a long way toward maintaining strong relationships.

2. **Stay connected:** Regularly check in with your support network, even when you are feeling well. Maintaining regular communication helps to strengthen your relationships and ensures that your network remains available when you need it.

3. **Be open and honest:** Share your feelings, concerns, and updates with your support network. Being open and honest about your experiences allows others to better understand your needs and offer appropriate support.

4. **Offer support in return:** Building a support network is a two-way street. Whenever possible, offer support and assistance to others in your network. Being there for others can strengthen your relationships and create a sense of reciprocity.

Remember, building a support network takes time, and it is okay to start small. Reach out to one person or join one support group, and gradually expand your network as you feel comfortable. Surrounding yourself with a supportive community can make a significant difference in your thyroid cancer journey, providing you with the strength and resilience to thrive.

Coping Strategies and Stress Management

Receiving a diagnosis of thyroid cancer can be overwhelming and stressful. It is normal to experience a range of emotions, including fear, anxiety, sadness, and anger. Coping with these emotions and managing stress is an essential part of your journey towards recovery and thriving after thyroid cancer. In this section, we will explore various coping strategies and stress management techniques that can help you navigate the challenges you may face.

Understanding Stress and Its Impact

Stress is a natural response to challenging situations, and a cancer diagnosis can undoubtedly be one of the most stressful events in a person's life. It is important to recognize that stress can affect both your physical and emotional well-being. Chronic stress can weaken the immune system, disrupt sleep patterns, and contribute to the development of other health issues. Therefore, finding effective ways to manage stress is crucial for your overall health and quality of life.

Coping Strategies

- **Seek Support:** Reach out to your support network, including family, friends, and support groups. Talking to others who have gone through similar experiences can provide comfort and reassurance. Consider joining a local or online support group specifically for thyroid cancer survivors. Sharing your feelings and concerns with others who understand can be incredibly helpful.

- **Educate Yourself:** Knowledge is power. Take the time to learn about thyroid cancer, its treatment options, and potential side effects. Understanding the disease and its management can help alleviate anxiety and empower you to make informed decisions about your health.

- **Practice Relaxation Techniques:** Engaging in relaxation techniques can help reduce stress and promote a sense of calm. Deep breathing exercises, meditation, yoga, and progressive muscle relaxation are all effective techniques that can be incorporated into your daily routine.

- **Maintain a Healthy Lifestyle:** Eating a balanced diet, getting regular exercise, and prioritizing sleep are essential for managing stress. Physical activity releases endorphins, which are natural mood boosters. Additionally, a healthy lifestyle can improve your overall well-being and help you cope better with the challenges of thyroid cancer.

- **Express Yourself:** Find healthy outlets for expressing your emotions. Journaling, painting, playing music, or engaging in any creative activity that resonates with you can be therapeutic. Expressing your feelings through art can provide a sense of release and help you process your emotions.

- **Practice Mindfulness:** Mindfulness involves being fully present in the moment and accepting it without judgment. Engaging in mindfulness exercises, such as mindful breathing or body scans, can help you stay grounded and reduce stress. By focusing on the present moment, you can let go of worries about the past or future.

- **Set Realistic Goals:** Setting realistic goals can give you a sense of purpose and control. Break down larger tasks into smaller, manageable steps. Throughout the process, be proud of your accomplishments, no matter how small they may seem. By setting achievable goals, you can maintain a positive outlook and boost your self-confidence.

- **Maintain a Positive Outlook:** Cultivating a positive mindset can make a significant difference in how you cope with thyroid cancer. Practice gratitude, surround yourself with inspiring people, and do things that bring you joy. Remember that your attitude and outlook can greatly impact your overall well-being.

Stress Management Techniques

1. **Exercise Regularly:** Physical activity is not only beneficial for your physical health but also for your mental well-being. Engaging in regular exercise can help reduce stress, improve mood, and boost your energy levels. Find activities that you enjoy, such as

walking, swimming, or dancing, and make them a part of your routine.

2. **Practice Time Management:** Feeling overwhelmed can contribute to stress. Learning effective time management techniques can help you prioritize tasks, set realistic deadlines, and reduce the feeling of being constantly rushed. Consider using tools such as calendars, to-do lists, or mobile apps to help you stay organized.

3. **Get Sufficient Rest:** Sleep is essential for your body's ability to heal and recover. Aim for seven to eight hours of quality sleep each night. Establish a relaxing bedtime routine, create a comfortable sleep environment, and limit exposure to electronic devices before bed to promote better sleep.

4. **Engage in Relaxing Activities:** Find activities that help you relax and unwind. This could include reading a book, taking a warm bath, listening to calming music, or practicing a hobby you enjoy. Engaging in activities that bring you peace and joy can help reduce stress and promote a sense of well-being.

5. **Seek Professional Help:** If you find that stress and anxiety are significantly impacting your daily life and well-being, do not hesitate to seek professional help. You can get the support and tools you need to effectively manage stress from a therapist or counselor.

They can also help you develop coping strategies tailored to your specific needs.

Remember, coping with thyroid cancer is a personal journey, and what works for one person may not work for another. It is essential to explore different coping strategies and stress management techniques to find what resonates with you. Be patient with yourself, practice self-care, and reach out for support when needed. With time and perseverance, you can develop effective coping mechanisms that will help you thrive after thyroid cancer.

Inspiring Stories of Thyroid Cancer Survivors

In this section, we will share inspiring stories of individuals who have successfully battled thyroid cancer and emerged as survivors. These stories serve as a testament to the strength, resilience, and determination of those who have faced this disease head-on. Each story is unique, but they all share a common thread of hope, courage, and the will to thrive.

Sarah's Journey to Empowerment

Sarah was diagnosed with thyroid cancer at the age of 32. Initially, she felt overwhelmed and scared, but she quickly realized that she had a choice - to let the diagnosis define her or to take control of her life. Sarah decided to embrace her journey and become an advocate for herself. She educated herself about thyroid cancer, treatment options, and the importance of self-care.

Throughout her treatment, Sarah maintained a positive mindset and surrounded herself with a strong support system. She found solace in connecting with other thyroid cancer survivors through support groups and online communities. Sarah's determination and resilience not only helped her navigate the challenges of treatment but also inspired others to take charge of their health.

Mark's Triumph over Adversity

Mark was diagnosed with an aggressive form of thyroid cancer at the age of 45. The news came as a shock to him and his family, but they refused to let fear consume them. After undergoing surgery, Mark received radioactive iodine therapy and external beam radiation. Despite the physical and emotional toll of treatment, Mark remained steadfast in his determination to overcome the disease.

Throughout his journey, Mark discovered the power of positivity and gratitude. He started a gratitude journal, where he wrote down three things he was grateful for each day. This practice helped him shift his focus from the challenges of cancer to the blessings in his life. Mark's story is a testament to the transformative power of a positive mindset and the importance of finding joy amid adversity.

Emily's Path to Self-Discovery

Emily was diagnosed with thyroid cancer at the age of 28. The diagnosis came at a time when she was already struggling with her sense of identity and purpose. Instead of letting cancer further derail her, Emily saw it as an opportunity for self-discovery and personal growth. She embarked on a journey of self-reflection and exploration, using her diagnosis as a catalyst for positive change.

During her treatment, Emily discovered the healing power of creativity. She started painting and writing as a way to express her emotions and find solace. Through her artwork, she found a sense of purpose and a newfound appreciation for life. Emily's story reminds us that even in the face of adversity, there is always room for personal growth and self-discovery.

Michael's Resilience and Determination

Michael was diagnosed with thyroid cancer at the age of 50. As a father of three, he knew he had to stay strong not only for himself but also for his family. Michael approached his diagnosis with unwavering determination and resilience. He underwent surgery, followed by radioactive iodine therapy and regular monitoring.

Throughout his treatment, Michael focused on maintaining a healthy lifestyle. He incorporated exercise into his daily routine and made conscious choices about his nutrition. By taking control of his physical health, Michael felt empowered and better equipped to face the challenges of cancer. His story serves as a reminder that small lifestyle changes can have a significant impact on overall well-being.

Lisa's Journey of Advocacy

Lisa was diagnosed with thyroid cancer at the age of 35. The diagnosis came as a shock, but Lisa refused to let it define her. She became an advocate for herself and others affected by thyroid cancer. Lisa started a blog where she shared her experiences, provided resources, and raised awareness about the disease.

Through her advocacy work, Lisa connected with numerous individuals who were going through similar experiences. She became a source of support and inspiration for others, offering guidance and a listening ear. Lisa's story highlights the power of advocacy and the importance of using our own experiences to make a positive impact on the lives of others.

These inspiring stories of thyroid cancer survivors remind us that a diagnosis does not define our destiny. With determination, resilience, and a supportive network, it is possible to overcome the challenges of thyroid cancer and thrive. Each survivor's journey is unique, but they all share a common thread of hope, courage, and the will to live life to the fullest.

Conclusion

The Thyroid Cancer Thriving Mindset

Receiving a thyroid cancer diagnosis can be frightening and overwhelming. However, with the right information, support system, and positive mindset, it is possible to not just survive but thrive in the face of this disease. This book has provided you with the knowledge and tools needed to understand your diagnosis, make informed treatment decisions, manage side effects, adopt healthy lifestyle habits, and cope with the emotional impact.

Remember that thyroid cancer is highly treatable, especially when caught early. Many people go on to live normal, full lives after treatment. Focus on the facets of health and life that you can control, such as eating nutrient-rich foods, reducing stress, connecting with supportive friends and family, and maintaining a hopeful outlook. Don't lose yourself in the world of cancer. You are still you, with dreams, interests, and bright days ahead.

Trust in your medical team, but also trust in your inner strength and resilience. Speak up when you have questions or concerns, and be an active participant in your healing journey. Thyroid cancer may have presented an unexpected challenge, but it does not define your future. You now have the knowledge and power to face whatever comes your way with courage, wisdom, and grace.

A thriving mindset chooses faith over fear, empathy over judgment, and meaning over despair. You are stronger than you know. With perseverance, passion, and purpose, you can triumph over thyroid cancer, transform your experience, and thrive on each new day. The end of this book is only the beginning of your next chapter. Go forward with hope.